Daniella Maria Soares de Oliveira
Marilis D. Miguel
Obdúlio G. Miguel

Isolation of verbascoside and validation of an analytical method

AF136812

Daniella Maria Soares de Oliveira
Marilis D. Miguel
Obdúlio G. Miguel

Isolation of verbascoside and validation of an analytical method

Method for standardizing the crude extract of the aerial parts of Buddleja stachyoides Cham. & Schltdl. (Scrophulariaceae)

ScienciaScripts

This book is a translation from the original published under ISBN 978-620-2-04817-0.

Publisher:
Sciencia Scripts
is a trademark of
Dodo Books Indian Ocean Ltd. and OmniScriptum S.R.L publishing group

120 High Road, East Finchley, London, N2 9ED, United Kingdom
Str. Armeneasca 28/1, office 1, Chisinau MD-2012, Republic of Moldova, Europe
Printed at: see last page
ISBN: 978-620-7-23823-1

SUMMARY

SUMMARY

In this work, a long-chain fatty acid, identified by NMR as triacontanoic acid, was isolated from the hexane fraction of the roots of *Buddleja stachyoides* Cham. & Schltdl. The compound identified as verbascoside, a glycosylated phenylpropanoid with pharmacological activities such as antioxidant, analgesic, anti-inflammatory and gastroprotective, was isolated from the ethyl acetate fraction of the aerial parts. A method using high-performance liquid chromatography was developed and validated to determine the content of verbascoside present in the crude alcoholic extract of the aerial parts of *B. stachyoides*. The analysis was carried out on a Phenomenex® Gemini-NX C18 analytical column (250 x 4.6 mm; 5 µm) using as mobile phase (pump A - aqueous solution with H_2SO_4 0.01 M, H_3PO_4 0.4% and $C_4H_{11}N$ 0.4%; pump B - (95:5) methanol: aqueous solution with H_2SO_4 0.05 M, H_3PO_4 2% and $C_4H_{11}N$ 0.2%; pump C - (90:10) Acetonitrile: aqueous solution with H_2SO_4 0.05 M, H_3PO_4 2%), DAD detector at 325 nm. The analytical method developed for determining the verbascoside marker proved to be reliable and suitable, as it met all the validation parameters required by RE No. 899 of May 29, 2003. This work is aimed at health professionals and researchers and offers them a contribution to the research, development and production chain of herbal medicines and pharmaceutical products based on extracts from *Buddleja stachyoides*, or any other plant species containing the substance verbascoside.

Keywords: *Buddleja stachyoides*. Scrophulariaceae. Analytical validation. Verbascoside. Phenylpropanoid. Antioxidant.

1 INTRODUCTION

Brazil is responsible for managing the largest biodiversity heritage in the world, with around 46,000 catalogued species, and has a long tradition of using medicinal plants, which has been passed down through generations (FLORA DO BRASIL, 2016). Despite the richness of the Brazilian flora, in the last twenty years the number of research studies on medicinal plants has only grown by 8% annually (FONSECA, 2012).

The plant species *Buddleja stachyoides* Cham. & Schltdl. belongs to the family Scrophulariaceae, (LOHMUELLER, 2012), known in Brazil as barbasco or verbasco, (FERREIRA, 1988), is used in home medicine based on popular tradition as an anti-haemorrhoidal, béquica (calms coughs), analgesic, sudorific, calming, emollient and anti-rheumatic. In animals, it is used to wash the eyes and treat bruises (wounds) in horses (MAHLKE, 2007; LORENZI, 2008). Ethnopharmacology records that tea made from the bark is used to treat lung ailments, while the roots are used against snakebite poisoning. The decoction of pieces of the whole plant in a liter of water is used in the form of baths, indicated in cases of contusions, bruises and pain in general. It grows spontaneously in pastures and vacant lots, where it is considered a weed (LORENZI, 2008). This species is native and not endemic to Brazil. Its phytogeographic domains are the Cerrado, the Atlantic Forest and the Pampas. In Brazil, its geographical distribution includes the Northeast (Bahia, Alagoas), Midwest (Federal District), Southeast (Minas Gerais, Espirito Santo, São Paulo, Rio de Janeiro), South (Paranà, Santa Catarina, Rio Grande do Sul) (SOUZA, 2010).

Substances from the *Buddleja* genus were isolated, such as: flavonoids (luteolin-7-O-glucoside), iridoids (acumbin, p- methoxycinnamoyl, buddlejoside A2, catalpol, methylcatalpol, vanillyljugol, feruloyljugol, buddjeloside A1), phenylethanoids, phenylpropanoids (verbascoside, isoverbascoside, leucosceptoside A and martinoside), sesquiterpenes

3

(buddledines A-E, dihydrobuddledine A, zerumbone, buddledone A-B, cyclochlorenone, hydroxycyclochlorenone), diterpenes (buddlejone, deoxybuddlejone, 11,14-dihydroxy-8,11,13-abietatrien-7-one, maitenone, crocetin monogentiobiosis ester) triterpenes (saikosaponin A; 45-48: buddlejasaponin 1-4; 49: mimengoside A; 50: mimengoside B, mixture of α-amyrin andβ-amyrin). (MAHLKE, 2007; HOUGHTON, 2003; VERTUANI et al., 2011; BACKHOUSE et al., 2008a).

The phenylpropanoid verbascoside [2-(3,4-dihydroxyphenletil)-1- O-α- L-ramnopyranosil-(1 -► 3)-β-D-(4-O-cafeyl)-glucopyranoside], also known as acteoside, is the main constituent of the crude alcoholic extract of the *B. stachyoides* species. (GITZEL FILHO et al., 2012). The biological properties of this substance have been described in the literature, and it has several activities, including antioxidant, anti-inflammatory, photoprotective and chelating. The anti-inflammatory activity of verbascoside was confirmed by an *in vitro* test carried out on primary human keratinocyte cell cultures, in which verbascoside was able to significantly reduce the release of pro-inflammatory chemokines in a dose-dependent manner. This study also demonstrated that it promotes the improvement and repair of inflammation in the skin, due to its reactive oxygen species (ROS) sequestering activity, antioxidant, iron chelating and glutathione transferase (GST) inducing properties. An *in vivo* study carried out on inflammation of the intestinal mucosa showed that it is able to inhibit the activation of pro-inflammatory proteins,

Consequently, the enzymatic activity of matrix metalloproteinase, the latter also involved in the phenomena of skin ageing. The results of this study suggest that verbascoside has the function of eliminating intracellular radicals, reducing the microscopic and macroscopic signs of colitis in rats. Thus, the administration of verbascoside may be beneficial in the treatment of inflammatory bowel disease (VERTUANI et al., 2011). Other studies have shown that verbascoside has antinociceptive activity, being more active than

4

ibuprofen (BACKHOUSE et al., 2008a), and also inhibits the enzyme prolyl oligopeptidase (POP), a protease that hydrolyzes small peptides with proline (GITZEL FILHO et al., 2012). The increase in neuroprotective effects and cognitive improvement with the use of POP inhibitors is notable. These substances are important for the treatment of clinical conditions such as neuropsychiatric disorders and neurodegenerative diseases (BORGES et al., 2010).

The interaction of verbascoside with phospholipid membranes was evaluated by a study in which a high affinity of this substance with the negatively charged membranes of phosphatidylglycerol (PG) compounds was observed, it promoted the phase separation of lipid domains in phosphatidylcholine (PC) membranes and formed a stable complex with the lipid (phospholipid/verbascoside). Despite its hydrophilic nature, the caffeoyl portion of verbascoside was located deep in the hydrophobic core of the PC membrane. It also altered the ionization behaviour of the PG phosphate group and interacted with the surface of the vesicles. The effects of verbascoside on the physical properties of membranes may help to explain some of its biological activities, such as antimicrobial and antioxidant activities (FUNES et al., 2010).

In other reports, mullein inhibited the enzymatic activity of angiotensin-converting enzyme, which may be beneficial against arterial hypertension, inhibited the formation of prostaglandin E2, tumor necrosis factor and nitric oxide and also suppressed the enzymatic activity of cyclooxygenase (COX-2). In a series of *in vitro* studies, it was clearly shown to have immunomodulatory, antiviral and anti-metastasis activity (LEE, WOO, AND KANG, 2005).

Due to its pharmacological interest, it is important to use a validated analytical method to quantify this component of the crude alcoholic extract of *B. stachyoides* that contains the verbascoside marker. This method could help

5

to standardize a herbal medicine made from the aerial parts of *B. stachyoides* and be used for dosage analysis in quality control.

The National Health Surveillance Agency (ANVISA), which regulates the registration and sale of herbal medicines in Brazil, has become increasingly demanding of pharmaceutical companies. Registration is possible once the safety and efficacy of herbal medicines have been proven through pre-clinical and clinical studies, literature data, simplified registration or traditional registration. Resolution RDC No. 26 of May 13, 2014, divided herbal medicines into two classes: herbal medicine and traditional herbal product. This last class of medicine was created by ANVISA in order to make it clear to the population whether the product used has undergone clinical tests of safety and efficacy or whether it has been approved for a period of safe and effective traditional use (BRASIL, 2014).

The validation of an analytical method for the determination of a marker is another requirement of the registration process and, in order for this method to generate reliable information about the sample, validation becomes a vital aspect for verifying analytical quality assurance (BARROS, 2002). There are several literatures in the field of chemical measurements and recommendations published by international and national bodies that require the validation of analytical methods (RIBANI et al., 2004). ANVISA published RDC No. 166 of July 24, 2017, which provides for the validation of analytical methods, replacing RE No. 899 of May 29, 2003, "Guide to the validation of analytical and bioanalytical methods". The analytical validation presented in this book was based on RE No. 899/2003, which was in force at the time of the validation. The parameters evaluated between the two legislations are similar, with RDC No. 166 being more rigorous in relation to statistical analysis (BRASIL, 2017).

Given the importance of this compound, the aim of this study was to isolate and identify the substance verbascoside from the ethyl acetate fraction, develop and validate a method for quantifying and standardizing the crude alcoholic extract of the aerial parts of *B. stachyoides*.

2 EXPERIMENTAL PART

2.1 COLLECTING PLANT MATERIAL

The plant material (aerial parts and roots) was collected at the Capâo do Cifloma, Federal University of Paranà, Jardim Botânico campus (25°26'53.7"S 49°14'15.8"W) in May and June 2011, when the research began.

The botanical identification of the species was carried out in the Herbarium of the Museu Botànico Municipal in the city of Curitiba, State of Paranà, compared with the exsiccate shown in figure 1 and registered under the number 339899 *Buddleja stachyoides* Cham. & Schltdl by the curator Osmar do Santos Ribas. The aerial parts and roots collected can be seen in figure 2.

The *B. stachyoides* species has authorization from the Brazilian Institute for the Environment and Renewable Natural Resources (IBAMA) for its morphoanatomical, chemical and biological evaluation, carried out in accordance with the resolution of the Genetic Heritage Management Council (CGEN) No. 35 of April 27, 2011.

FIGURE 1 - PHOTOGRAPH OF *Buddleja stachyoides* EXSICATA COLLECTION No. 339899

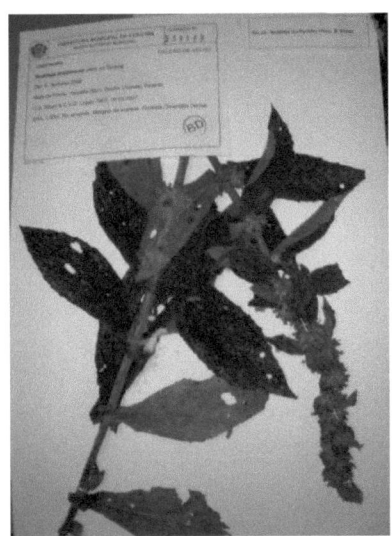

SOURCE: OLIVEIRA (2011)

FIGURE 2 - PHOTOGRAPH OF EXAMPLES OF THE PLANT SPECIES *Buddleja stachyoides*

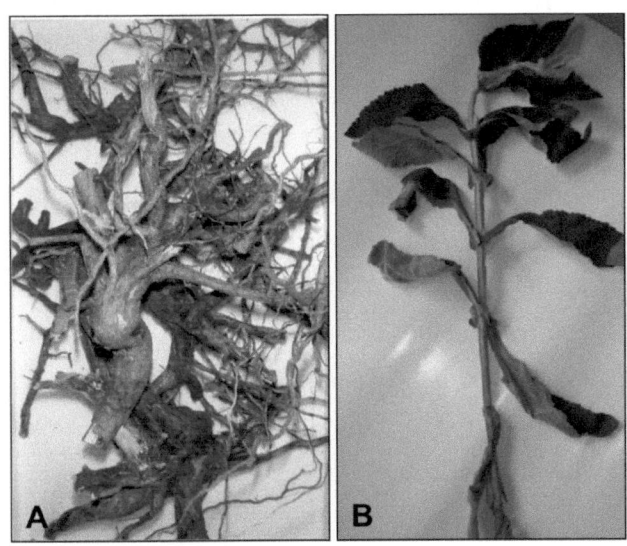

SOURCE: OLIVEIRA (2012)

LEGEND: A: roots; B: aerial parts

2.2 EQUIPMENT

The precipitate was purified using a Gilson® high-performance liquid chromatography system with DAD 171 and ELSD TMII detectors, a model 322 pump and a Luna® PFP C18 preparative chromatography column with a length of 250 mm, an i.d. of 21.20 mm and a particle size of 5 µm. and 5 µm particle size, and the Waters® high performance liquid chromatography system model PDA 996, with ELSD 2420 detector and Luna® PFP C18 analytical chromatography column 250 mm long, 4.6 mm i.d. and 5 µm particle size.

The nuclear magnetic resonance (NMR) experiments were carried out on two Bruker spectrometers® model 600 MR and Avance® III HD 600, operating at 14.1 T, observing the nuclei of ^{1}H and ^{13}C at 600.13 and 150.90 MHz respectively, equipped with a 5 mm quadrinuclear inverse probe with z gradient. All chemical shifts were observed in relation to the TMS signal at 0.00 ppm as an internal reference or in relation to the solvent signal. The ^{1}H and ^{13}C {^{1}H} spectra were acquired with a spectral window of ~11 ppm and ~240 ppm, respectively.The H-^{113}C single bond (HSQC) and long distance (HMBC) correlation NMR spectra were optimized for average coupling constants ^{1}J(H,C) and^{LR}J(H,C) of 140 and 8 Hz, respectively.

To validate the analytical method, a Merck-Hitashi® high performance liquid chromatography system was used, with pump model L7100, solvent degasser model L7812; automatic injector model L-7200; DAD detector model L7455; L7000 interface connected to the Windows Professional operating system and Phenomenex® Gemini-NX C18 analytical chromatography column, 250 mm long, 4.6 mm d. i. and 5µm particle size.i. and 5 µm particle size, serial number 462569-14.

2.3 EXTRACTION

From the dried, stabilized and crushed plant, 5.97 and 2.39 kg of the aerial parts and roots were weighed, respectively. They were then extracted separately in a Soxhlet apparatus in accordance with the patent (PI 0601703-

7A) (CARVALHO, 2001).

The dried plant material was placed in the glass holder of the Soxhlet apparatus (containing a porous plate and a layer of cotton). About 8000 mL of 96 °GL ethanol was added to this system for extraction. A ball condenser and a round-bottomed flask containing glass beads were connected to the modified Soxhlet apparatus (with tap). This system was heated in a heating mantle. After the heating started, the extract liquid contained in the flask evaporated and condensed at 60°C in the ball condenser, running through the plant material again. When the extract meniscus in the side channel of the Soxhlet reached the reflux point, the extract was discharged into the flask by siphoning and the process was repeated approximately 10 times until the liquid contained in the side channel of the Soxhlet was clear. This procedure avoids thermal degradation of the substances contained in the flask, as the amount of extracting liquid is constant in the system and is capable of solvating the compounds (CARVALHO, 2001). Due to the large quantity of aerial parts, the extraction procedure was carried out three times and then they were mixed.

After extraction, the crude alcoholic extracts (aerial parts and roots) were obtained and then used to obtain the fractions and isolates. The analytical validation was carried out only with the crude extract of the aerial parts, due to the greater ease of obtaining the standard and the pharmacological activities related to the verbascoside marker.

2.4 OBTAINING FRACTIONS

The fractions were obtained using the liquid-liquid partitioning method with solvents (P.A.) of different polarities: n-hexane, chloroform, ethyl acetate, using a soxhlet apparatus connected to a ball condenser and a flat-bottomed flask with glass beads. The system was heated in a heating mantle and left to reflux for around 12 hours. During the partitioning process, a quantity of distilled water was added to the crude alcoholic extract to facilitate the

11

separation of the solvents, resulting in a remaining fraction.

2.5 YIELD OF CRUDE EXTRACTS AND FRACTIONS

After extraction and liquid-liquid partitioning, the extracts and fractions were concentrated in a rotaevaporator and then evaporated to dryness in a water bath at 60°C. The yields of the crude extracts and fractions were calculated as a percentage in relation to the amount of dry starting plant material used in the extraction and the weight of the samples after drying.

2.6 DEVELOPMENT OF ANALYTICAL METHODOLOGY

To find a phytochemical marker in the species and help identify the compounds, two HPLC methods were developed, using the following as the mobile phase: [pump A: aqueous solution consisting of $H2SO4$ (0.01 M), $H3PO4$ (0.4%) and $(C2H5)2NH$ (0.4%); pump B: methanol: aqueous solution consisting of $H_2 SO_4$ (0.05 M), $H3Po4$ (2%) and $(C2H5)2NH$ (0.2%); in a ratio of 90:10, respectively; pump C: acetonitrile: aqueous solution consisting of $H2So4$ (0.05 M) and $H3Po4$ (2%), in a ratio of 90:10, respectively]; sample dilution: methanol and diluent phase ($H2o$ + 2% $H3Po4$). Under the following analysis conditions: wavelength 325 nm; oven temperature 35 °C; injection volume 40 µL. In the first method, the samples were injected with the crude alcoholic extract and fractions of the aerial parts using the mobile phase gradient described in Table 1.

TABLE 1 - GRADIENT OF ELUIATION OF THE FIRST ANALYTICAL METHOD DEVELOPED IN HPLC FOR THE ANALYSIS OF THE GROSS EXTRACT AND FACTIONS OF THE AERIAL PARTS OF Buddleja stachyoides

TIME (min)	PHASE A (%)	PHASE B (%)	PHASE C (%)	FLOW (mL/min)
0,0	98,0	0,0	2,0	1,2
5,0	98,0	0,0	2,0	1,2
6,0	95,0	3,0	2,0	1,2
8,0	82,0	16,0	2,0	1,2
15,0	70,0	16,0	14,0	1,2
35,0	57,0	16,0	27,0	1,2

53,0	34,0	64,0	2,0	1,2
58,0	34,0	64,0	2,0	1,2
60,0	10,0	88,0	2,0	1,2
69,0	10,0	88,0	2,0	1,2
70,0	98,0	0,0	2,0	1,2
80,0	98,0	0,0	2,0	1,2

SOURCE: oLIvEIRA (2012)

In the second method, only the crude alcoholic extract of the aerial parts and the verbascoside standard were injected under the same conditions as the first, but with some alterations as shown in Table 2.

TABLE 2 - ELUCTION GRADIENT OF THE SECOND ANALYTICAL METHOD DEVELOPED IN HPLC FOR THE ANALYSIS OF THE RAW EXTRACT OF THE AERIAL PARTS OF *Buddleja stachyoides*

TIME (min)	PHASE A (%)	PHASE B (%)	PHASE C (%)	FLOW (mL/min)
0,0	100	0	0	1,1
3,0	100	0	0	1,2
5,0	90	7	3	1,2
15,0	81	16	3	1,2
28,0	70	21	9	1,2
36,0	70	21	9	1,2
40,0	59	26	15	1,2
45,0	59	26	15	1,2
47,0	20	65	15	1,2
53,0	20	65	15	1,2
54,0	100	0	0	1,1
60,0	100	0	0	1,1

SOURCE: OLIVEIRA (2012)

2.7 ISOLATION AND IDENTIFICATION

2.7.1. Purification of fractions

The fractions were purified using column chromatography with silica gel 60 Merck® stationary phase (0.063 - 0.200 mm). Around 10 g of each fraction (hexane, ethyl acetate) was incorporated into the silica gel to form a pellet. This pellet was subjected to column chromatography, where the sample was

13

eluted using a solvent passage system with increasing polarity gradients, starting with 100% n-hexane P.A., then a mixture of hexane and ethyl acetate P.A. in the ratio 70:30, using ethyl acetate as the polarity gradient and increasing the interval every 5% until 100%. Next, the mixture of ethyl acetate and methanol P.A. was used in the ratio 90:10, using methanol as a polarity gradient and increasing the interval every 5% up to 100%. The fractions were collected in small vials of approximately 10 mL, which were then exposed to room temperature to allow the solvents to evaporate.

2.7.2. Purification of isolates

During the purification of the hexane fraction of the roots, 144 aliquots were collected. The vials that had started to precipitate were washed with petroleum ether, left in the fridge for 5 minutes and then centrifuged to separate the precipitate. From vials 49 to 59, 8.5 mg of precipitate was obtained, which was named FHR1 and its structure identified by NMR at [13] C and H.[1]

In the purification of the ethyl acetate fraction from the aerial parts of *B. stachyoides,* 107 aliquots were collected and during the drying process, 3 vials showed signs of crystallization, which were centrifuged and pooled, obtaining a precipitate. This precipitate was resuspended in methanol and chromatographed on a silica chromatoplate, using ethyl acetate, ferric acid and water (90:0.5:0.5) as the mobile phase and 2-aminoethylester diphenylboric acid in ethanol as the developer. The separated bands were scraped off and placed in vials, dissolved in methanol and centrifuged to remove the silica. The result was 10 mg of the compound called FAEPA1, which was analyzed by hydrogen nuclear magnetic resonance, but was not pure. A second purification was carried out using preparative HPLC chromatography, where 10 mg were dissolved in 300 μL of DMSO and 300 μL were injected using the following method: [Mobile phase: FA - H_2O + 0.1% H3PO4, FB - ACN + 0.1% H3PO4; time 0-20 minutes (80-FA:20-FB), time

20-27 minutes (75-FA:25-FB), time 27 minutes (0-FA:100-FB); flow 24 ml/min]. A third purification was carried out using an HPLC analytical column, 1.2 mg were dissolved in 300 μL of methanol, with which injections of 50 and 100 μL were made, manually recovering the main peak. The method used: [Mobile phase: FA - H2O + 0.1% H3PO4, FB - ACN + 0.1% H3PO4; time 0-20 minutes (80- FA:20-FB), time 22-29 minutes (0-FA:100-FB), time 30 minutes (80- FA:20-FB); flow 1.0 mL/min]. After this purification, 0.4 mg of the component was recovered with a purity of 99.93% (HPLC) and identification was carried out by NMR-[1] H and one- and two-dimensional techniques, at CD3OD and room temperature.

The verbascoside standard was isolated from the ACOEt fraction of *Duranta vestita* Cham. leaves, Verbenaceae. This fraction was purified using a Merck® silica gel 60 column, for which a pellet was prepared with 5 parts silica to 1 part fraction. The sample was then eluted with a mixture of solvents, starting with 100% n-hexane P.A., using ACOEt as the polarity gradient and increasing the interval every 10% up to 100%. Next, a mixture of ACOEt and MeOH P.A. was used in the ratio 90:10, using MeOH as the polarity gradient and increasing the interval from 10% to 100% of the same, then water was used as the gradient, with an interval from 50% to 100% of H2O. Vials 49 to 90 were collected and injected into a C18 preparative column (HPLC) using the following method: mobile phase A: H2O + 0.1% H_3PO_4 and mobile phase B: MeOH; gradient: time 0-7 minutes (85 to 80%-FA:15 to 20%-FB) and time 8-32 minutes (35%-FA:65%-FB). The isolated substance appeared as a beige powder, with a purity of 99.89% (HPLC) and its structure identified by NMR from [13] C and [1] H. (CANTELI, 2012).

2.8 VALIDATION OF THE ANALYTICAL METHOD FOR QUANTIFICATION of the verbascoside marker

The second analytical method (table 2) was chosen for analytical validation and quantification of the verbascoside marker present in the crude extract of the aerial parts of *B. stachyoides*. The concentration of verbascoside in the sample was calculated using the L7000 interface system connected to Windows Professional (Merck-Hitashi equipment), taking into account the peak area found, the equation of the line and the actual dilution factors [Concentration (mg/g) = Area x Dilution factor x Equation of the line (scalar)].

The parameters evaluated in the validation of the analytical method for the dosage of verbascoside were: specificity, linearity, precision by repeatability, intermediate precision, accuracy and robustness, in accordance with RE No. 899 of May 29, 2003, drawn up by ANVISA.

The analytical curve was prepared with the standard solution of verbascoside, isolated from the ethyl acetate fraction of *Duranta vestita* Cham. leaves (Verbenaceae), at a concentration of 0.30 mg/mL in methanol. Five concentrations dissolved in the diluent phase were prepared from this solution (0.08 mg/mL; 0.09 mg/mL; 0.10 mg/mL; 0.11 mg/mL; 0.12 mg/mL) and injected in triplicate.

Precision by repeatability was carried out with 6 determinations at 100% of the test concentration to check the agreement between the results within a short period of time with the same analyst and the same instrumentation. Intermediate precision was also carried out with 6 determinations at 100% of the test concentration and served to check the agreement between the results of the two analysts, in the same laboratory, but obtained on different days. In this test, the samples were diluted 1:250 to remain within the analytical curve.

The accuracy parameter used the standard addition method, in which known quantities of the verbascoside standard were added to the crude alcoholic extract. The study was carried out at 3 concentrations, low, medium and high in the range of the analytical curve, in triplicate, totaling 9 tests. To obtain the low concentration close to the theoretical one (0.083 mg/mL), 125 µL of the crude alcoholic extract sample were added 1:50, 100 µL of the verbascoside standard (0.30 mg/mL) and 775 µL of diluent phase. To obtain the average concentration close to the theoretical one (0.107 mg/mL), 125 µL of the 1:50 crude alcoholic extract sample, 180 µL of the verbascoside standard (0.30 mg/mL) and 695 µL of diluent phase were added. To obtain the high concentration close to the theoretical one (0.119 mg/mL), 125 µL of the 1:50 crude alcoholic extract sample, 220 µL of the verbascoside standard (0.30 mg/mL) and 655 µL of diluent phase were added. Accuracy was calculated as the percentage recovery of the known quantity of the analyte added to the sample and the acceptance criterion is 95 to 105%. (BRASIL, 2003).

For the robustness parameter, the stability analysis of the solution was carried out; the same sample used for the repeatability accuracy parameter was injected 24 hours after its preparation. Other ways of assessing the robustness of the method were to dilute mobile phase A (1:2), with a consequent change in pH from 2.0 to 3.0 and also to change the oven temperature to 40°C.

3 RESULTS

3.1 YIELD OF CRUDE EXTRACTS AND FRACTIONS

The weight of the starting dry plant material from the aerial parts was 5970 g. After extraction and concentration (in a rotary steamer and water bath at 60°C until dry), 797.64 g of crude alcoholic extract was obtained, with a yield of (13.36 ± 2.34)% in relation to the starting dry material. To obtain the crude extract of the roots, 2385 g of the dried starting plant material was weighed. After extraction and concentration (in a rotary evaporator and water bath at 60°C until dry), 62.48 g of crude alcoholic extract was obtained, with a yield of (2.62 ± 0.056)% compared to the dry starting material. From these extracts, 40.57g of the crude alcoholic extract of the aerial parts and 3.68g of the crude alcoholic extract of the roots were taken to carry out the biological activities; the rest was used for fractionation. Table 3 shows the yield of the fractions in relation to the amount of crude alcoholic extract used.

TABLE 3 - YIELD OF FRACTIONS AND CRUDE ALCOHOLIC EXTRACTS

SAMPLE	AIR PARTS		ROOTS	
	MASS (g)	INCOME (%)	MASS (g)	INCOME (%)
Alcoholic extract Gross	757,07	-	58,80	-
Hexane fraction	102,20	13,50	10,52	17,89
Chloroform fraction	54,77	7,23	11,97	20,36
Fraction Acetate Ethyl	82,05	10.84	2,05	3,49
Fraction Hydroalcoholic Remaining	518,05	68,43	34,26	58,26

SOURCE: OLIVEIRA (2012)

3.2 DEVELOPMENT OF ANALYTICAL METHODOLOGY

The chromatograms of the fractions and crude extract of the aerial parts obtained through the first analytical method developed to select a phytochemical marker in the plant species *B. stacyoides*, showed a predominant peak with a retention time similar to the verbascoside pattern, which can be seen in figure 3. Although the method separated the major peak, it did not show good resolution.

FIGURE 3 - MULTICHROMATOGRAMS OF THE CRUDE EXTRACT AND FRACTIONS OF THE AERIAL PARTS OF *Buddleja stachyoides*

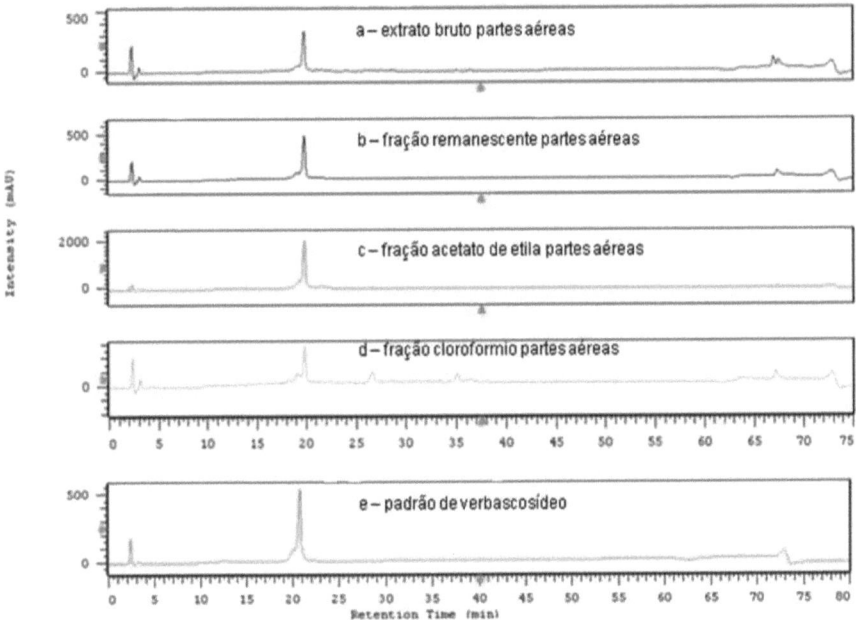

SOURCE: oLivEiRA (2012)

LEGEND: a - crude extract of aerial parts; b - remaining fraction of aerial parts; c - ethyl acetate fraction of aerial parts; d - chloroform fraction of aerial parts; e - verbascoside pattern

After developing the second HPLC method, the samples were injected with the crude alcoholic extract of the aerial parts, the crude alcoholic extract of the aerial parts co-injected with the verbascoside standard and the verbascoside standard. The chromatograms are shown in figure 4. The chromatogram obtained from the crude alcoholic extract of the aerial parts

19

showed a major peak with an intensity of approximately 450 mAU, at a retention time of 32.61 minutes. The chromatogram of the crude alcoholic extract of the aerial parts co-injected with the verbascoside standard showed a major peak at a retention time of 32.53 minutes with an intensity of approximately 1650 mAU and the chromatogram of the verbascoside standard showed a peak at a retention time of 32.69 minutes with an intensity of approximately 1400 mAU. The retention times of the major peak were practically the same in the three samples, demonstrating that there is a similarity between the peak present in the crude alcoholic extract and the verbascoside peak.

The UV spectra and the purity of the peaks obtained for the samples of the crude alcoholic extract of the aerial parts, the crude alcoholic extract of the aerial parts added to the verbascoside standard and the verbascoside standard can be seen in figure 5. The UV spectra of the three samples are very similar, with absorption at 329.1 nm and peak purities greater than 99%. For the peak of the crude extract of the aerial parts the purity obtained was 99.95%, for the peak of the crude extract of the aerial parts added to the verbacoside standard the purity obtained was 99.93% and for the peak of the verbascoside standard the purity was 99.89%.

The spectral correlations of the peaks shown in figure 6 for the samples of the crude extract of the aerial parts and the crude extract of the aerial parts plus the verbascoside standard were checked by comparing them with the vebascoside standard in the HPLC library. All the correlations were greater than 95%, demonstrating the existence of similarity between the UV spectra. For the crude alcoholic extract of the aerial parts added to the verbascoside standard, the spectral correlation was 99.73%, which was higher than the spectral correlation found (95.05%) for the crude extract of the aerial parts.

FIGURE 4 - CHROMATOGRAMS OF THE CRUDE EXTRACT OF THE AERIAL PARTS AND

CODEO VERBS PATTERN

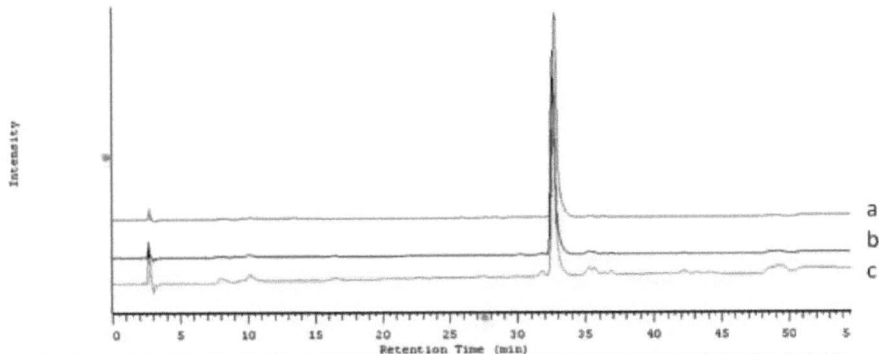

SOURCE: OLIVEIRA (2012)

LEGEND: a - chromatogram of the crude extract of the aerial parts; b - chromatogram of the crude extract of the aerial parts co-injected with the verbascoside standard; c - chromatogram of the verbascoside standard

FIGURE 5 - UV SPECTRA AND PEAK PURITY OF THE RAW ALCOHOLIC EXTRACT OF THE AIR PARTS AND VERBASCOSiDEO PATTERN

21

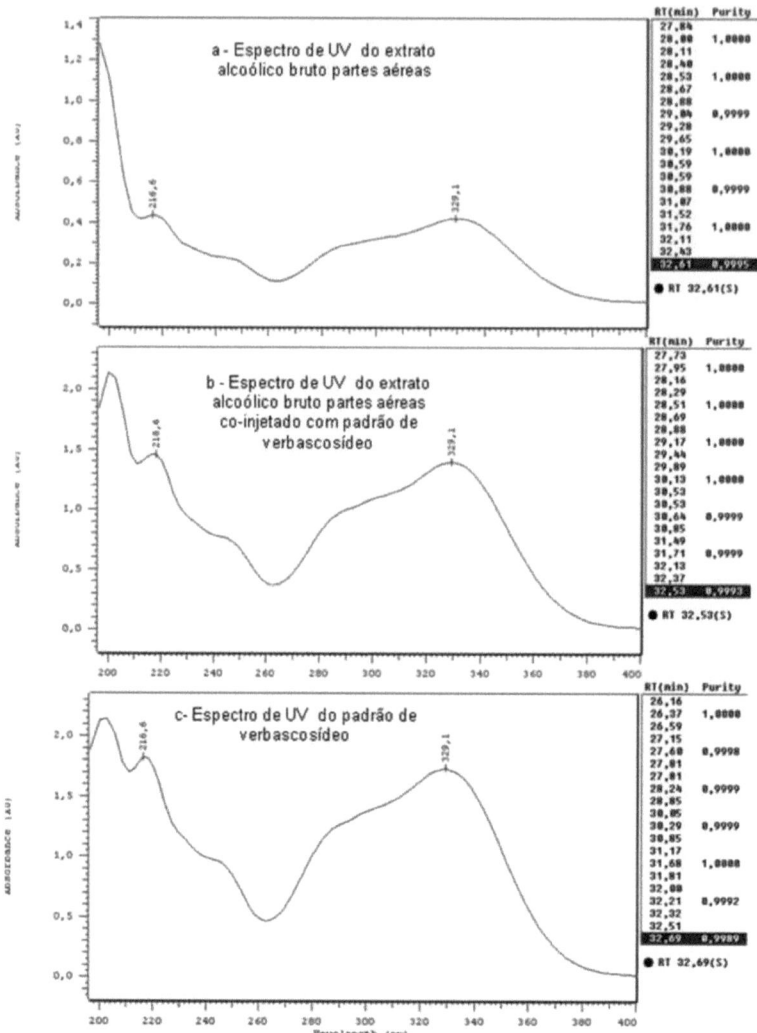

SOURCE: OLIVEIRA (2012)

LEGEND: a - UV spectrum and peak purity of the crude extract of the aerial parts; b - UV spectrum and peak purity of the crude extract of the aerial parts contaminated with verbascoside standard; c - UV spectrum and peak purity of the verbascoside standard

FIGURE 6 - SPECTRAL CORRELATION OF THE SAMPLES WITH THE VERBASCOSIDEO PATTERN

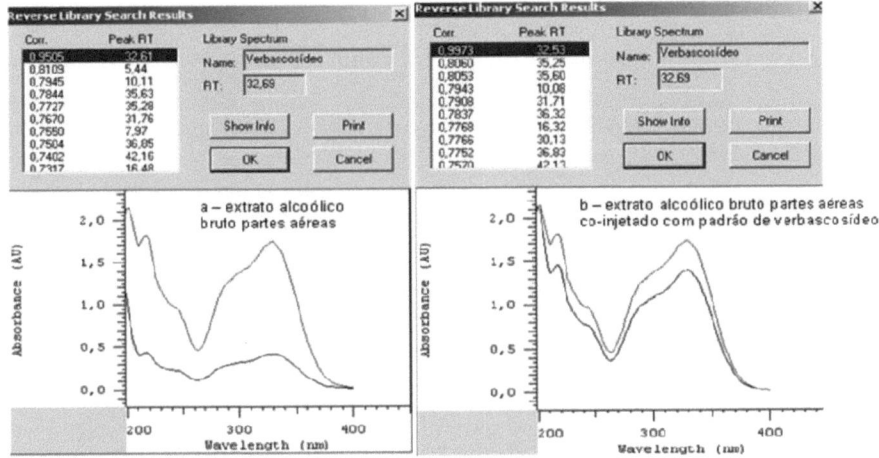

SOURCE: OLIVEIRA (2012)

LEGEND: a - spectral correlation of the sample of crude alcoholic extract of aerial parts; b - spectral correlation of the sample of crude alcoholic extract of co-injected parts with verbascoside pattern

3.3 ISOLATION AND IDENTIFICATION

The compound FHR1 isolated from the hexane fraction of the roots of *B. stachyoides* appeared as white amorphous crystals soluble in chloroform. After NMR analysis at[1] H and[13] C, it was identified as a long-chain fatty acid, with a structure similar to that of triacontanoic acid ($C_{30}H_{60}O_2$, figure 7), also known as melissic acid.

FIGURE 7 - CHEMICAL STRUCTURE OF COMPOUND FHR1 IDENTIFIED AS TRIACHONANOIC ACID

SOURCE: OLIVEIRA (2017)

The NMR spectrum of[1] H, shown in figure 8, shows a triplet in the region of 0.88 ppm, with a coupling constant of J = 6.9 Hz, indicating the presence of a long carbon chain with a terminal CH3. There is also a multiplet at 1.26 ppm.

23

Considering that the signal at 0.88 ppm is equivalent to three hydrogens, the signals were integrated and the signal at 1.26 ppm resulted in 42 hydrogens, i.e. 21 CH2s in a similar chemical environment. There are also two more multiplets at 1.62 and 2.03 ppm and a triplet at 2.34 ppm (J = 7.4 Hz), which represent three more CH2, information that matches the integrals and the region of the spectrum in which the signals appear. The signal at 5.35 ppm indicates the presence of OH from the carboxylic acid.

FIGURE 8 - RMN SPECTRUM FROM[1] H OF COMPOUND FHR1 (600 MHZ, cDCl3, 20° C)

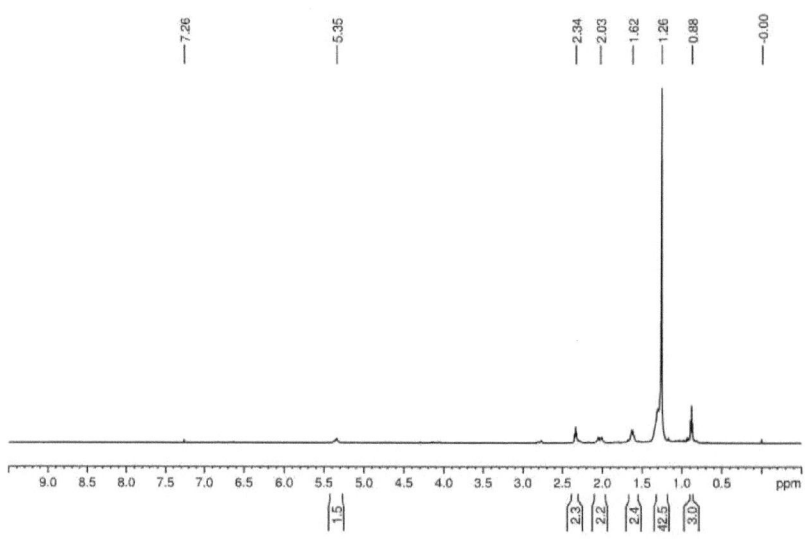

SOURCE: OLIVEIRA (2017)

The NMR spectrum of[13] C, shown in figure 9, shows the presence of six signals. The first, at 14.1 ppm, corresponds to the terminal CH3 carbon. The signals between 22.7 and 34.1 ppm correspond to the long-chain CH2 carbons. The signal at 179.7 ppm indicates the presence of an acid carbonyl, which suggests that there is a carboxylic acid function at one end of the carbon chain.

FIGURE 9 -[13] C RMN SPECTRUM OF COMPOUND FHR1 (150.90 MHZ, CDC | 3, 20° C)

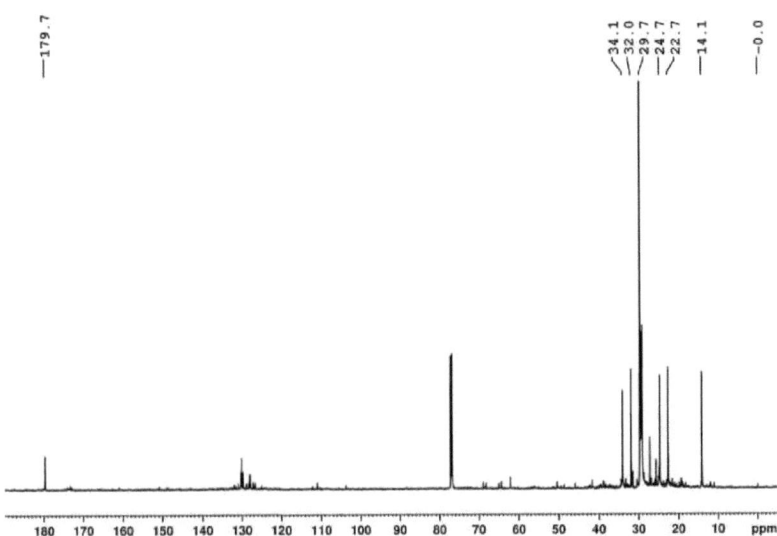

SOURCE: The author (2017)

The chemical shift signals and the coupling constants (J) obtained from the NMR spectra of[1] H and NMR of[13] C of the FHR1 compound were compared with the literature described in table 4, and even though the solvents are different, the signals are very similar, indicating that this is the same compound.

TABLE 4 - COMPARISON OF THE RMN-[1] H AND RMN-[13] C SIGNALS OF COMPOUND FHR1 WITH THE LITERATURE

POSITION	TYPE OF C	COMPOSITE FHR1				(MACEDO, 2011)		
		RMN-[1] H (600 MHZ, CDCl3)		RMN-[13] C (150.90 MHZ, CDCl3)		NMR-[1] H (300 MHz, C5D5N)		NMR-[13] C (75 MHz, C5D5N)
		δ (PPm)	TYPE, J (Hz)	δ (ppm)		δ (PPm)	J (Hz)	TYPE, J (Hz)
1	CH3	0,88	t, J=6.9	14,1		0,89	t, J=6.0	14,2
2	CH2	1,62	m	22,7		1,41	m	22,9
3	CH2	1,26	m	24,7		1,29	m	25,6
4-27	CH2	1,26	m	29,7		1,29	m	29,6
28	CH2	2,03	m	32,0		1,82	m	29,8

25

| 29 | CH2 | 2,34 | t, J=7.4 | 34,1 | 2,54 | t, J=7.4 | 34,9 |
| 30 | COOH | - | - | 179,7 | - | - | 175,9 |

SOURCE: OLIVEIRA (2017)

Triacontanoic acid has already been isolated from other plants such as *Hibiscus tiliaceus* L., *Eucalyptus globulus*, Senna *cearensis* and *Senna martiana* (MELECCHI, 2005; FREIRE, 2005; FERREIRA et al., 2009; MACEDO, 2011). Ferreira et al. (2009) isolated and identified a high content of triacontanoic acid in the hexanic extract of the stem of *Senna cearensis* which, in addition to other properties, has antithrombotic and antiplatelet activity. According to the study by Pan et al. (2012) *Vitis thunbergii* demonstrated various cardioprotective effects that can be modulated through its identified compounds, such as: β-sitosterol, β-sitosterol-3-O-β-D-glucoside, ampelopsin C, betulinic acid, botulinum, caffeic acid, friedelin, heyneanol A, 1-dotriacontanol, lupeol, luteolin-7-O-glucoside, miyabenol A, narcissin, oligostilbenes, piceatanol, quercetin-3-O- galactoside, quercitrin, rutin, stigmasterol, triacontanoic acid, vanillic acid, viniferin, viniferal, vitisin A, vitisin C and vitisinols AD. Therefore, triacontanoic acid may be important in the treatment and prevention of cardiovascular diseases, particularly atherosclerosis, due to its antiplatelet activity.

The compound FAEPA1 isolated from the ethyl acetate fraction of the aerial parts of *B. stachyoides*, after the first purification on chromatoplate, was injected into the HPLC and the major peak appeared in 9.5 minutes (figure 10), after which it was collected and cut into four parts, as shown in figure 11. Proton NMR was carried out on the 4 tubes in order to mix the pure fractions that corresponded to the same compound. The tubes mixed were 7, 8 and 9, obtaining 1.2 mg, but in the end the compound was still not completely pure.

FIGURE 10 - CHROMATOGRAM OF THE COMPOUND OBTAINED IN HPLC

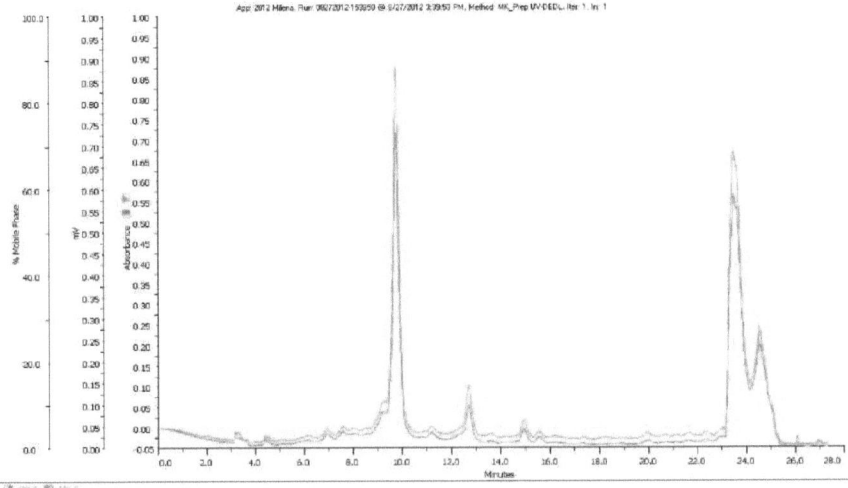

To continue the purification of the compound, a third purification was carried out using an HPLC with an analytical column. The chromatograms obtained and the UV spectrum are shown in figure 12. The first chromatogram (a) represents the ELSD presence detector, and the second (b) refers to the UV detector. After the second purification, 0.4 mg of the apparently pure compound was recovered.

FIGURE 11 - PEAK OF THE COMPOST CUT AND COLLECTED IN FOUR PARTS

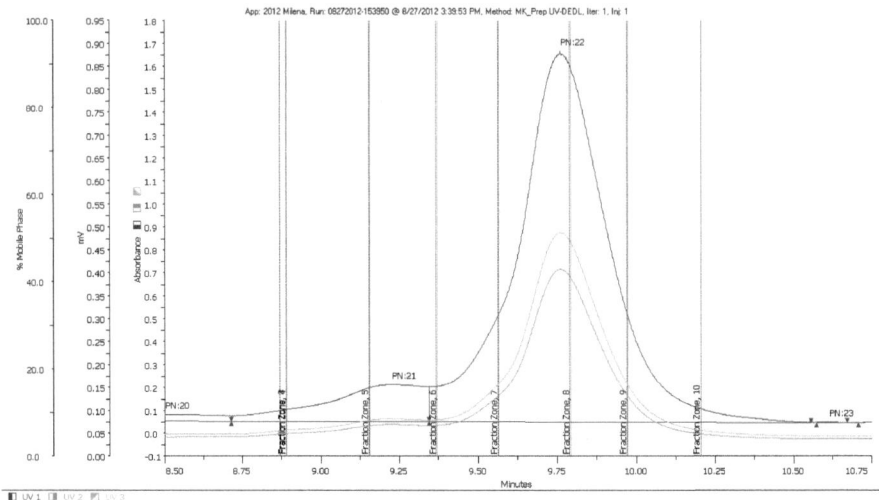

FIGURE 12 - CHROMATOGRAMS AND UV SPECTRUM OF THE COMPOUND OBTAINED IN HPLC

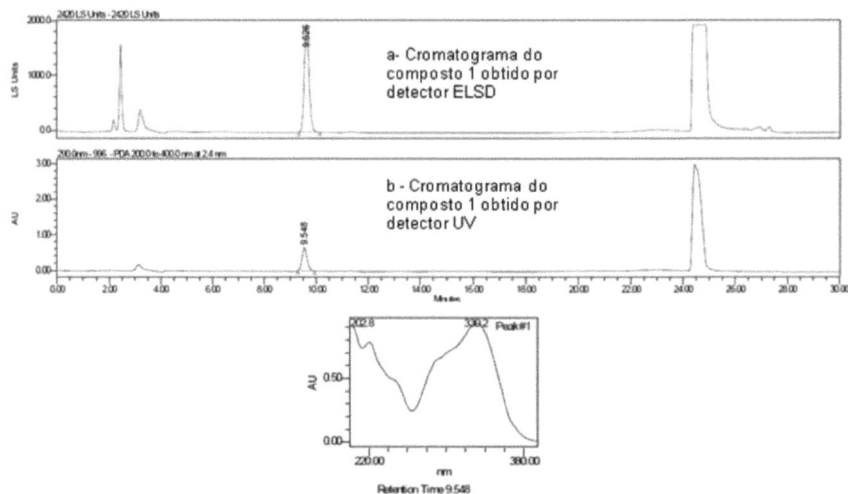

Compound FAEPA1 appeared as white amorphous crystals and was soluble in methanol. After NMR analysis at^1 H, it was identified as a verbascoside glycosylated phenylpropanoid (C H O$_{293615}$, figure 13).

The comparison of the signals, chemical shift and coupling constant (J)

obtained from the projection of the[13] C NMR and[1] H NMR spectra of the FAEPA1 compound with the values obtained in the literature for the verbascoside is shown in Table 5. These tests, together with the HSQC and HMBC assignment, enabled the caffeic ring, the sugars (glucose and rhamnose) and the phenylethanoid ring to be found.

The NMR-[1] H spectrum of the compound shows the presence of a set of signals at δ 6.66 (1H, d, J = 7.89 Hz, H-5), δ 6.69 (1H, d, J = 2.02 Hz, H-2) and δ 6.56 (1H, dd, J = 7.89 Hz, J = 2.02 Hz, H-6), and another set at δ 6,77 (1H, d, J = 8.07 Hz, H-5" '), 6.96 ppm (1H, dd, J = 8.25 Hz, J = 2.2 Hz, H-6" ') and 7.06 ppm (1H, d, J = 2.02 Hz, H-2" '). These resonances are characteristic of the presence of two 1,3,4-trisubstituted aromatic systems. One of these aromatic systems is part of a caffeoyl moiety due to the signals from two olefinic protons at δ 6.28 (1H, d, J = 15.77 Hz, H-8" ') and δ 7.60 (1H, d, J = 15.77 Hz, H- 7" '), which indicates a trans geometry. Proton signals at δ 2.80 (2H, m, H-7), 3.71 ppm (1H, m, H-8a) and δ 4.05 (1H, m, H-8b) revealed that the second aromatic system is part of the phenylethanoid portion. The NMR-[1] H spectrum also showed a number of signals between 3.00 and 4.00 ppm, suggesting the existence of sugar in the molecule. A signal at δ 1.08 (3H, d, J = 6.24 Hz, H-6") is observed for the 3H of the CH3 group corresponding to rhamnose and, in addition, a signal at δ 5.18 (1H, d, J = 1.47 Hz, H-1") with a small coupling constant can be assigned to the anomeric proton of an α-L-ramnose. O

FIGURE 13 - PROTON SPECTRUM FOR COMPOUND FAEPA1

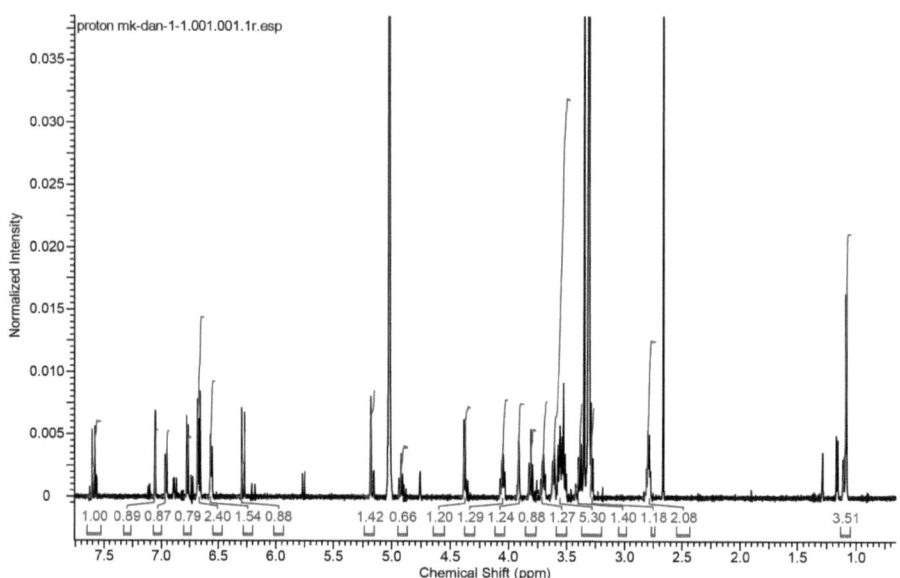

anomeric proton signal appears for glucose (β-hexopyranose) at δ 4.38 (1H, d, J = 7.89 Hz, H-1').

To obtain the projection of the carbons of the molecule corresponding to each proton, the Heteronuclear Single Quantum Correlation (HSQC) technique was used, which correlates heteronuclear coupling (proton-carbon) spaced by bond ($^1 J$) at short distances (figure 14). The quartenary carbons and the carbonyl were determined using the Heteronuclear Multiple Bond Correlation (HMBC) technique, which correlates heteronuclear coupling spaced by several bonds ($2J$ or$^3 J$), which is important for establishing correlations H-[113] C through two and three bonds (figure 15). The presence of the carbonyl by the HMBC was detected by the correlation of the 7.60 proton with a 166.5 ppm carbon.

FIGURE 14 - HETERONUCLEAR SINGLE QUANTUM CORRELATION (HSQC) TECHNIQUE USED FOR COMPOUND FAEPA1

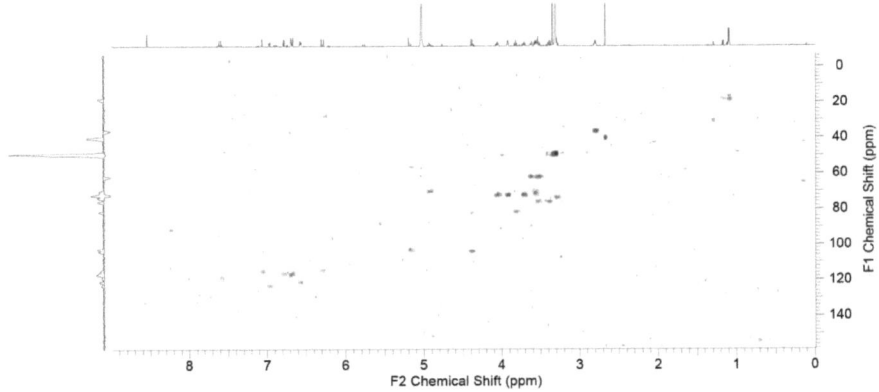

FIGURE 15 - HETERONUCLEAR MULTIPLE BOND CORRELATION (HMBC) TECHNIQUE USED FOR COMPOUND FAEPA1

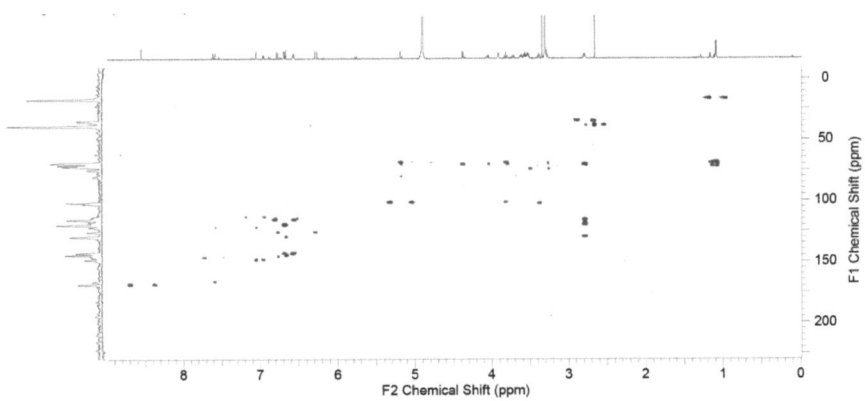

The structure of compound FAEPA1 is shown in figure 16.

FIGURE 16 - STRUCTURE OF COMPOUND FAEPA1

SOURCE: OLIVEIRA (2012)

TABLE 5 - COMPARISON OF THE NMR-[1] H AND PROJECTED NMR-[13] C VALUES OBTAINED FOR THE ISOLATED COMPOUND AND THE VALUES FIND IN THE LITERATURE FOR VERBASCOSiDEO

Position	(GITZEL FILHO et al., 2012) NMR[1] H - Verbascoside			Isolated compound NMR H[1]			(ESCALONA, 2006) 1H- NMR Verbascosideo		
	Type of C	δ (ppm)	J (Hz)	NMR [13] C δ (ppm)	δ (ppm)	J (Hz)	NMR [13] C δ (ppm)	δ (ppm)	J (Hz)	NMR [13] C δ (ppm)
caffeic										
1'''	C	-	-	127,7	-	-	125,8			125,5
2'''	CH	7,07	d (2,0)	115,3	7,06	d (2,02)	114,8	7,06	d (1,9)	114,7
3'''	C			146,87			145,5			145,5
4'''	C			149,82			148,4			148,5
5'''	CH	6,79	d (8,2)	116,56	6,77	d (8,07)	116,2	6,78	d (8,2)	113,3
6'''	CH	6,97	dd (8.2; 2.0)	123,26	6,96	dd (8.25; 2,2)	123	7	dd (8.2; 1,9)	121,4
7'''	CH	7,6	d (15,9)	148,06	7,6	d (15,77)	148,1	6,2	d (15,9)	145,7
8'''	CH	6,28	d (15,9)	114,74	6,28	d (15,77)	114,2	7,6	d (15,9)	115,4
9'''	C=O			168,35			166,5			166
phenylethanoid										
1	C			131,52			129,7			131,5
2	CH	6,71	d (2,0)	117,16	6,69	d (2,02)	117,2	6,72	-	117,1
3	C			146,16			144,7			146
4	C			144,71			143,1			144,8
5	CH	6,69	d (8,1)	116,36	6,66	d (7,89)	116,2	6,68	d (8,0)	116,3
6	CH	6,58	d (8,1)	121,3	6,56	dd (7,89;2,2)	120,9	6,57	dd (8;2)	121,2
7	CH₂	2,8	m	36,6	2,8	m	36,4	2,79	t	36,5
8	CH₂	4,05 - 3,75	m	72,3	4,05 - 3,71	m	72,1	3,79 - 3,70	m	72,1
Glucose										
1'	CH	4,39	d (7,90)	104,23	4,38	d (7,89)	103,9	4,38	d (7,9)	104,1
2'	CH	3,4	d (9,2;	76,24	3,39	t (8,4)	76	3,39	dd (9; 7,9)	77,7

32

			7,9)							
3'	CH	3,81	t(9,2)	81,7	3,81	t (9,17)	81,4	3,81	t (9,0)	84,5
4'	CH	4,93	m	70,46	4,92	m	70,2	4,98	t (9,5)	70
5'	CH	3,56	m	76,07	3,56	m	71,3	3,79	-	75,5
6'	CH_2	3,71 - 3,56	m	62,41	3,61 - 3,52	m	62,1	3,6	dd (11.5; 1,4)	62,6
Rhamnose										
1"	CH	5,2	d (2,0)	103,07	5,18	d (1,47)	102,7	5,18	d (1,3)	102,7
2"	CH	3,93	m	72,39	3,92	dd (3,3; 1,83)	72	3,92	dd (3.0;1.7)	72,2
3"	CH	3,59	m	72,09	3,56	m	71,3	3,6	-	72,2
4"	CH	3,32	m	73,83	3,29	t (9,5)	73,7	3,29	t (9,5)	73,9
5"	CH	3,59	m	70,64	3,56	m	71,3	3,6	-	70
6"	CH3	1,1	d (6,2)	18,49	1,08	d (6,24)	18,5	1,09	d (6,2)	17,9

SOURCE: OLIVEIRA (2012)

The biological properties of verbascoside, also known as acteoside, have been described in the literature, and it has various activities, including antioxidant, anti-inflammatory, photoprotective and chelating. From the ethyl acetate fraction of *B. officinalis* flowers, the compounds luteolin and verbascoside were isolated, which showed potent antioxidant activity (PIAO, 2003).

Lee, Woo, and Kang (2005) also evaluated the compound verbascoside isolated from *B. officinalis,* which showed an inhibition in the enzymatic activity of the angiotensin-converting enzyme and could be beneficial in cases of arterial hypertension. A series of *in vitro* studies clearly indicate that it has immunomodulatory, antiviral and anti-metastasis activity. Verbascoside had a protective effect against liver toxicity induced by CCl_4 in mouse liver and decreased the levels of nitrite generated in the decomposition of nitric oxide (NO). It was also reported that this compound inhibited the formation of prostaglandin E2, tumor necrosis factor alpha (TNF-α) and nitric oxide, as well as suppressing the enzymatic activity of cyclooxygenase (COX-2).

In the study by Backhouse et al. (2008a), the compounds luteolin and luteolin-7-O-glucoside, isolated from *B. globosa,* suppressed inducible nitric oxide synthase (iNOS) and COX-2, enzymes responsible for the production of nitric oxide and the release of PGE_2 , which, respectively, show increased expression in human tissue tumors (HU; KITTS, 2004). Luteolin has been shown to reduce lipopolysaccharide (LPS) levels and completely suppress the formation of PGE_2 (HARRIS et al., 2006). Luteolin-7-O-glucoside showed moderate inhibition of thromboxane and leukotriene synthesis, resulting in anti-inflammatory activity, as well as demonstrating antioxidant activity (ODONTUYA et al., 2005).

The analgesic effect of *B. globosa* was evaluated by Backhouse et al. (2008a) using the abdominal writhing test with intraperitoneal injection of acetic acid. The animals were treated with the different extracts (at doses of 200, 100, 50 and 25 mg/kg), verbascoside (0.05 mmol/kg) and Ibuprofen (0.07 mmol/kg) and the average effective doses, i.e. those that produced 50% antinociception (ED50) were calculated for each extract and reference drug. The results obtained were: ethanolic extract (effect: 79.8 ± 14%) and (ED50: 53.5 ± 6.0 mg/kg); methanolic (effect: 85.5 ± 4.2%) and (ED50: n.d); Ibuprofen (effect: 50 ± 4.1%) and (ED50: 14.4 ± 4.3 mg/kg) and verbascoside (effect: 67.6 ± 2.3%) and (ED50: n.d); luteolin-7-o-glucoside (effect: 27.0 ± 9.1%) and (ED50: n.d) and showed that verbascoside was more active than ibuprofen and almost twice as active as luteolin in the writhing test.

Backhouse et al. (2008b) also evaluated the methanolic extract of *B. globosa*, at a dose of 600 mg/kg, which showed anti-inflammatory activity orally (61.4%) and topically (56.7%) and analgesic action orally (38.5%), relating these effects to the isolated compounds verbascoside (1.8%) and lutein 7-o-glucoside (1.1%). The interaction of verbascoside with phospholipid membranes was evaluated by Funes (2010), who observed a significant affinity of this substance for the negatively charged membranes of phosphatidyl glycerol (PG) compounds, promoting phase separation of the lipid domains in phosphatidylcholine (PC) membranes, forming a stable complex with the lipid (phospholipid/verbascoside). Despite its hydrophilic nature, the caffeoyl portion of the verbascoside was localized deep in the hydrophobic core of the PC membrane. It also altered the ionization behaviour of the PG phosphate group and interacted with the vesicle surface. The presence of verbascoside decreased particle size in unilamellar PG vesicles by increasing the area of the phospholipid headgroup. A localization of verbascoside was proposed, filling the upper region of the PG in the bilayers close to the phospholipid/water interface. The effects of verbascoside on the physical properties of membranes may help to explain some of its biological activities, such as antimicrobial and antioxidant activities (FUNES, 2010).

The methanolic extract of *B. crispa* showed significant antioxidant and inhibitory activity on the 5-lipoxygenase enzyme (AHMAD, 2008).

Vertuani et al. (2011) observed the very significant antioxidant effect of verbascoside using various determination methods. In addition, the anti-inflammatory activity of verbascoside was confirmed by an *in vitro* test carried out on primary human keratinocyte cell cultures, in which verbascoside was able to significantly reduce the release of pro-inflammatory chemokines in a concentration-dependent manner. This study also demonstrated that it promotes the improvement and repair of inflammation in the skin, due to its reactive oxygen species (ROS) sequestering activity, antioxidant, iron chelating and glutathione transferase (GST) inducing properties. The *in vivo* study, conducted on inflammation of the intestinal mucosa, showed that verbascoside is able to inhibit the activation of pro-inflammatory proteins and, consequently, the enzymatic activity of matrix metalloproteinase, the latter also being involved in skin ageing phenomena. The results of this study suggest that verbascoside has the function of eliminating intracellular radicals, reducing the microscopic and macroscopic signs of colitis in rats, making its administration beneficial in the treatment of inflammatory bowel disease (VERTUANI et al., 2011).

The study by Liu et al. (2003) showed that verbascoside has a protective effect against the increase in free radical levels during plasma lipid peroxidation, and its administration protects membranes from damage, reducing the level of oxidative stress. The redox potential of verbascoside, as an electron donor, protects cells against cytotoxicity and apoptosis and is mediated by glucose oxidase (CHIOU et al., 2004). This preventive potential may be important in the treatment of diseases caused by oxidative stress, such as gastric ulcers induced by acidified ethanol (KIM et al., 2005).

The crude extract of *B. brasiliensis* Jacq. ex Spreng, fractions and the compound verbascoside were evaluated for their inhibition of the enzymes: acetylcholinesterase (AChE), dipeptidyl peptidase IV (DPP-IV) and prolyl oligopeptidase (POP). The compound showed a significant inhibition of POP in a dose-dependent manner with an IC value$_{50}$ of (1.3 ± 0.2) µM, similar to that of the positive control, baicalin, with an IC_{50} of (1.2 ± 3) µM. (GITZEL FILHO et al., 2012). The enzyme prolyl oligopeptidase (POP) is a protease that hydrolyzes small peptides with proline. The use of POP inhibitors increases neuroprotective effects and promotes cognitive improvement (BORGES et al., 2010). These compounds are important for the treatment of clinical conditions such as neuropsychiatric disorders and neurodegenerative diseases (GITZEL FILHO et al., 2012).

3.4 VALIDATION OF THE ANALYTICAL METHOD FOR QUANTIFICATION of the verbascoside marker

The analytical curve of the verbascoside standard was linear in the intended working range with a coefficient of determination (r^2) of 0.9869, which is higher than the specification for phytotherapics of 0.98, as shown in figure 17.

After obtaining the analytical curve, it was possible to calculate the concentration of verbascoside present in the sample of crude alcoholic extract of the aerial parts. We weighed 134 mg of the crude alcoholic extract sample (equivalent to 1 g of dried plant drug, as 797.64 g of dried crude alcoholic extract was obtained from 5970 g of dried starting plant material) and diluted it in a 50 mL volumetric flask with methanol, after which this solution was diluted 1:5 in the diluent phase, giving a final dilution of 1:250. The concentration found was 21.47 mg/g of verbascoside in relation to the dry plant drug, as shown in figure 18. The sample was diluted to fit the analytical curve according to the calculation: 21.47 mg/ 250 mL = 0.085 mg/mL final concentration of verbascoside.

FIGURE 17 - LINEARITY CURVE WITH THE VERBASCOSiDEO PATTERN

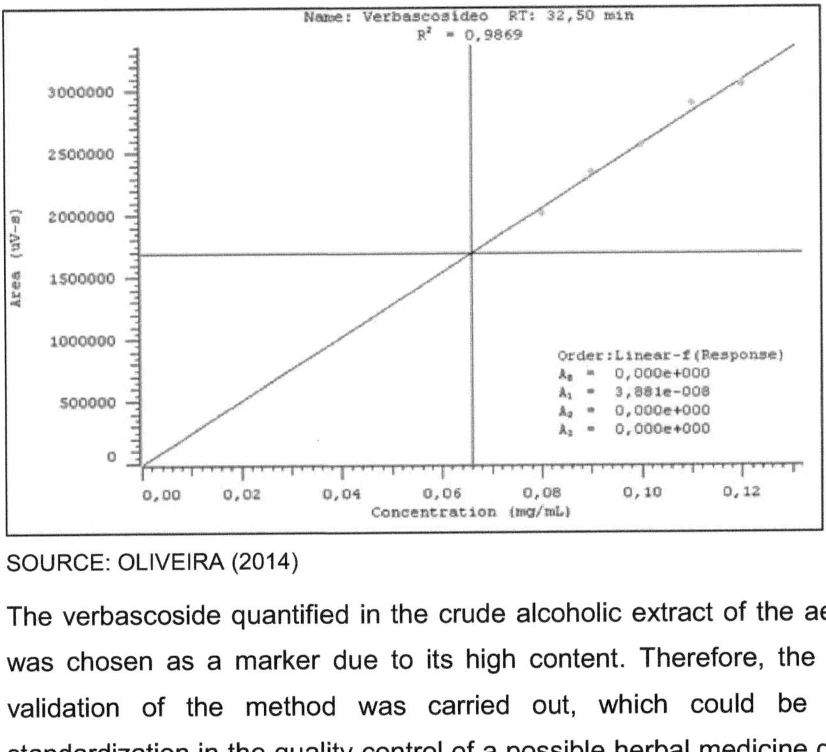

SOURCE: OLIVEIRA (2014)

The verbascoside quantified in the crude alcoholic extract of the aerial parts was chosen as a marker due to its high content. Therefore, the analytical validation of the method was carried out, which could be used for standardization in the quality control of a possible herbal medicine developed with the aerial parts of *Buddleja stachyoides*.

FIGURE 18 - CONCENTRATION OF VERBASCOSIDEO IN THE RAW ALCOHOLIC EXTRACT OF THE AIR PARTS OF *B. stachyoides*

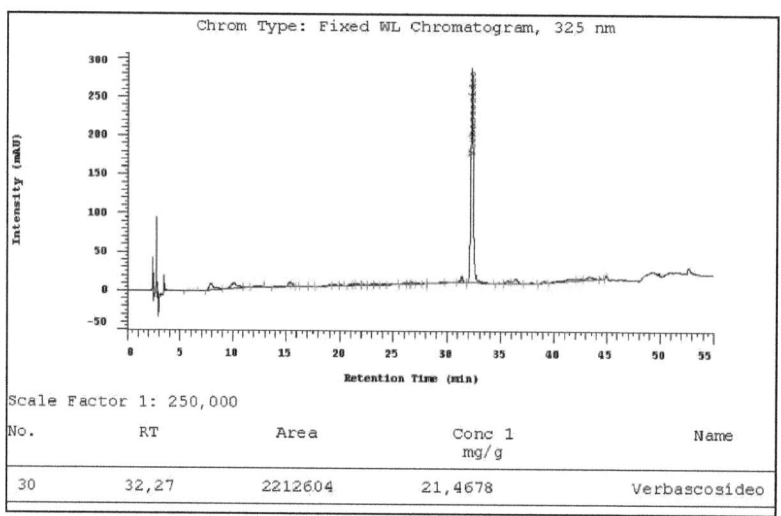

Chrom Type: Fixed WL Chromatogram, 325 nm

Scale Factor 1: 250,000

No.	RT	Area	Conc 1 mg/g	Name
30	32,27	2212604	21,4678	Verbascosideo

SOURCE: OLIVEIRA (2014)

The influence of the solvent ethyl alcohol hydrated from cereals 96 °GL was evaluated through the specificity test, which showed no peak with the same retention time as the verbascoside or any spectral similarity with the standard. This proved that the solvent used in the extraction did not contain any component that could interfere with the detection of verbascoside.

Figure 19 shows the UV spectrum with absorption at 329.1 nm. The purity of the verbascoside peak (99.88%), present in the crude alcoholic extract of the aerial parts, is higher than the 99% specification. The spectral comparison between the verbascoside peak of the sample and the verbascoside standard showed a spectral correlation of 99.96%, indicating the existence of similarity between the UV spectra and the same chromatographic profile, as shown in figure 20.

FIGURE 19 - UV SPECTRUM, PURITY AND SPECTRAL CORRELATION OF THE VERBASCOSIDEO PEAK PRESENTED IN THE RAW ALCOHOLIC EXTRACT OF THE AIR PARTS OF *B. stachyoides*

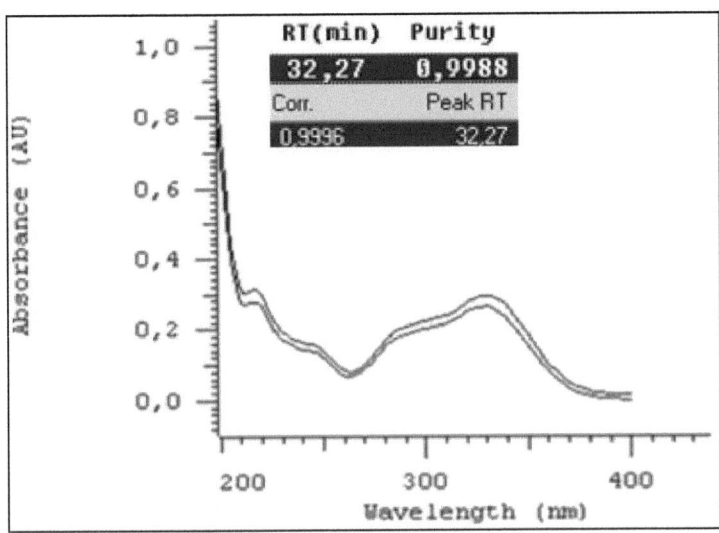

SOURCE: OLIVEIRA (2014)

FIGURE 20 - CHROMATOGRAPHY PROFILE (*FINGERPRINT*) OF THE RAW ALCOHOLIC EXTRACT OF THE AIR PARTS OF *B. stachyoides* AND THE WORKING PATTERN of VERBASCOSIDE

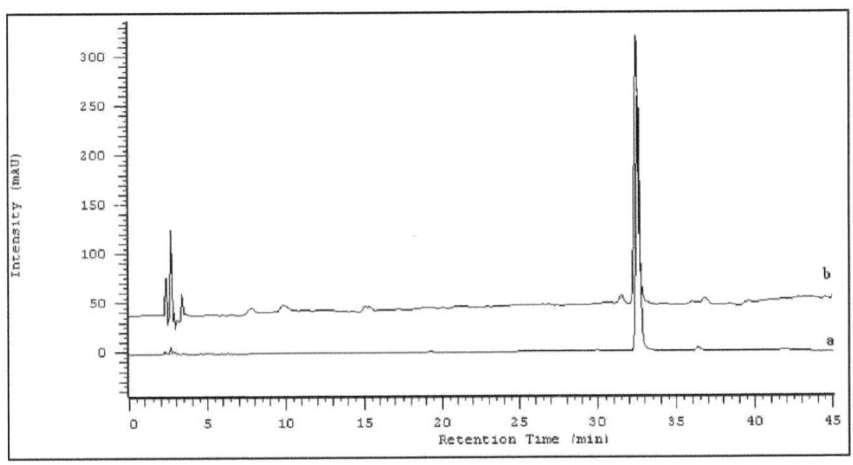

SOURCE: OLIVEIRA (2014)

LEGEND: a: Verbascoside reference standard; b: crude alcoholic extract

Accuracy by repeatability for analyst 1 showed a relative standard deviation (RSD%) between the 6 injections of 0.87% and an average concentration of

21.44 mg/g. Analyst 2 showed an average concentration of 20.57 mg/g and a relative standard deviation of 0.41%; these results are within the specified limits (RSD ≤ 5%). In intermediate precision, the average concentration between the two analysts was 21.01 mg/g with a relative standard deviation of 2.26%, which is within the specified limits (RfD ≤ 5%). These results confirm that the proposed method is reproducible.

In the accuracy test, practical concentrations of 0.083, 0.105 and 0.116 mg/mL were found, and when compared with the theoretical concentrations, recovery rates of 100.72%, 98.32% and 97.81% were obtained for the low, medium and high concentrations, respectively.

Therefore, the proposed method was accurate, as the recovery rates of the added standard remained within the 95% to 105% range. (BRASIL, 2003).

In the robustness test, the solution stability parameter showed a verbascoside content of 20.92 mg/g with a relative standard deviation of 0.28%, compared to the average of the intermediate precision, indicating that the sample remains stable, with little change in content after 24 hours of preparation. With regard to the pH parameter and the composition of the mobile phase, when diluting mobile phase A 1:2, in addition to changing the composition of the mobile phase, there was also a change in pH (which used to be around 2.0 and in this analysis was around 3.0). A verbascoside concentration of 20.45 mg/g was obtained, with a relative standard deviation of 1.81%. For the oven temperature parameter, the concentration found was 20.59 mg/g with a relative standard deviation of 1.41%. The three parameters proved to be robust for the proposed method, as all the relative standard deviations were lower than the specified limit (RSD ≤ 5%). Table 6 shows the results obtained in the analytical validation of the method for quantifying verbascoside.

Validation is a dynamic and constant process that must begin with the planning of the analytical strategy and continue throughout its development and transfer (BARROS, 2002). The analytical method must be revalidated

40

whenever changes occur in the process, equipment, sample standardization, procedure or when it is used again after a certain period of time. International and national standards and quality systems emphasize the importance of validating analytical methods and documenting the validation work in order to obtain reliable results that are suitable for their intended use (RIBANI et al., 2004).

The analytical method developed for the determination of the verbascoside marker, a major compound present in the crude extract of the aerial parts of *B. stachyoides,* proved to be reliable and adequate, as it met all the parameters required by Resolution - RE n° 899, of May 29, 2003. This method could help standardize the marker in quality control if a drug is developed from the aerial parts of *B. stachyoides in the* future.

TABLE 6- RESULTS OF THE VALIDATION OF THE ANALYTICAL METHOD FOR THE quantification of verbascoside in the crude extract of the aerial parts of *buddleja stachyoides*

ANALYZED PARAMETER		SPECIFICATION	RESULTS
Specificity	Influence of the excipient	Cannot interfere with the assay of the analyte	No interference from ethyl alcohol 99.88%
	Peak purity Correlation with standard peak	Min.99%	99,96%
		Min.95%	Samples with the same
	Fingerprint	Samples with the same chromatographic profile	chromatographic profile
Linearity	Analytical curve	$r^2 \geq 0.98$	$r^2 = 0.9869$
Precision	Repeatability	Analyst 1 : DPR ≤ 5%	0,87%
	Intermediate	Analyst 2: DPR ≤ 5%	0,41%
		DPR ≤ 5%	2,26%
Accuracy	Pattern Addition	95 to 105% recovery	100,72%
			98,32%
			97,80%

Robustness	Solution stability pH and FM composition Oven temperature	DPR ≤ 5%	0,28%
			1,81%
			1,41%

SOURCE: OLIVEIRA (2014)

LEGEND: DPR: Relative Standard Deviation; r^2 = coefficient of determination; FM: mobile phase

4 CONCLUSION

This work isolated the compound FHR1, a long-chain fatty acid, obtained from the purification of the hexane fraction of the roots of *Buddleja Stachyoides* and identified as the possible structure of triacontanoic acid. From the ethyl acetate fraction of the aerial parts, the compound FAEPA1 was isolated, identified as the phenylpropanoid verbascoside, the major compound of the species, which has pharmacological activities cited in the literature as antioxidant, analgesic, anti-inflammatory, gastroprotective and POP inhibitor. The analytical method developed and validated for the quantification of verbascoside and standardization of the crude alcoholic extract of the aerial parts proved to be reliable, sensitive, precise, reproducible, simple and low-cost, as well as meeting all the validation parameters required by ANVISA RE No. 899 of 29 May 2003. It is therefore of great importance in the research, development and production chain of herbal medicines and pharmaceutical products based on extracts from *Buddleja Stachyoides*, or any other plant species containing the substance verbascoside.

REFERENCES

BARROS, C. B. **Rev Biológico**, v. 64, p. 175, 2002.

BACKHOUSE, N.; DELPORTE, C.; APABLAZA, C.; FARiAS, M.; GOÏTY, L.; ARRAU, S.; NEGRETE, R.; CASTRO, C.; MIRANDA, H. Antinociceptive activity of *Buddleja globosa* (matico) in several models of pain. **J Ethnopharmacol**, v. 119, p. 160-165, 2008a.

BACKHOUSEA, N.; ROSALES, L., APABLAZA, C.; FARIAS, M.; GOÏTY, L.; ERAZO, S.; NEGRETE, R.; THEODOLUZ, C.; RODRiGUEZ, J.; DELPORTE, C. Analgesic, anti-inflammatory and antioxidant properties of *Buddleja globosa*, Buddlejaceae. **J Ethnopharmacol**, v. 116, p. 263269, 2008b.

BORGES, N. S.; DALCOL, I. GITZEL FILHO, A.; RIVERO, A. C.; ADOLPHO, L. O.; MARIN, D. F. Phytochemical and enzymatic activity study of Artemisia verlotorum Lamotte. Jornada acadêmica integrada, Universidade Federal de Santa Maria, Anais 25ª , 2010.

BRAZIL. National Health Surveillance Agency - ANVISA. Collegiate Board Resolution - RDC No. 26, of May 13, 2014. Provides for the registration of herbal medicines and the registration and notification of traditional herbal products. Available at: <http://portal.anvisa.gov.br/documents/33836/351410/Consolidado+de+norm mas+da+COFID+%28Vers%C3%A3o+V%29/3ec7b534-a90f-49da-   9c53-ce32c5c6e60d> Accessed on: 07 May 2017.

BRAZIL. National Health Surveillance Agency - ANVISA. Resolution RE n° 899 of May 29, 2003. Guide to the validation of analytical and bioanalytical methods. Available at: <http://portal.anvisa.gov.br/documents/10181/2718376/RE_899_2003_C OMP.pdf/ff6fdc6b-3ad1-4d0f-9af2-3625422e6f4b> Accessed on: 11 Mar. 2013.

BRAZIL. National Health Surveillance Agency - ANVISA. Resoluçâo da

Diretoria Colegiada - RDC n° 166, 24/07/2017, Dispoe sobre validaçâo de métodos analiticos. Available at: <http://portal.anvisa.gov.br/documents/10181/2721567/RDC_166_2017_COMP.pdf/d5fb92b3-6c6b-4130-8670-4e3263763401> Accessed on: 13/12/2017.

CANTELI, V. C. D.; **Phytochemical composition and biological activities of *Duranta vestita* Cham., Verbenaceae.** Dissertation (Master's Degree in Pharmaceutical Sciences) - Health Sciences Sector. Federal University of Paranà, Curitiba, 2012.

CARVALHO, J. L. de C. **Contribution to the phytochemical and analytical study of *Nasturtium officinale* R. BR., Brassicaceae.** 88f. Dissertation (Master's Degree in Pharmaceutical Sciences) - Health Sciences Sector, Federal University of Paraná. Curitiba, 2001.

CHIOU, W. F.; LIN, L. C.; CHEN, C. F. Acteoside protects endothelial cells against free radical-induced oxidative stress. **J Pharm Pharmacol**, v. 56, p. 743-748, 2004.

ESCALONA, C. D. R. A. **Study of the chemical standardization and evaluation of the topical analgesic activity of an active extract of *Buddleja globosa* Hope, Buddlejaceae, matico.** 77f. Dissertation (degree in Pharmaceutical Chemistry) - Department of Pharmacological and Toxicological Chemistry, Department of Pharmacology, University of Chile, Santiago, 2006.

FERREIRA, H. D. **Taxonomic revision of the species of Buddleja L. (Buddlejaceae) occurring in Brazil.** 111 f. Dissertation (Master's Degree in Plant Biology) - Campinas Institute of Biology, State University of Campinas, São Paulo, 1988.

Botanical Garden of Rio de Janeiro. Available at: <http://floradobrasil.jbrj.gov.br/>. Accessed on: May 22, 2017.

FONSECA, M. C. M. **Epamig researches the production of medicinal plants for use in the SUS**. Space for the producer. Viçosa, 2012.

FUNES, L.; LAPORTA, O.; CERDAN-CALERO, M.; MICOL, V.; **Chem Phys Lipids**, v. 163, p. 190, 2010.

GITZEL FILHO, A.; MOREL, A. F.; ADOLPHO, L.; ILHA, V.; GIRALT, E.;TARRAGÓ, T.; DALCOL, I. !.inhibitory effect of Verbascosideo isolated from *Buddleja brasiliensis* Jacq. ex Spreng on prolyl oligopeptidase activity. **Phytother Res**, v. 10, n. 26, p. 1472-1475, oct. 2012.

HARRIS, G. K.; QIAN, Y.; LEONARD, S. S.; SBARRA, D. C.; SHI, X. Luteolin and chrysin differentially inhibit cyclooxygenase-2 expression and scavenge reactive oxygene species but similarly inhibit prostaglandin E2 formation RAW 264.7 cells. **J Nutr**, v.136, p.15171521, 2006.

HOUGHTON, P.J.; MENSAH, A. Y.; IESSA, N.; HONG, L. Y. Terpenoids in Buddleja: relevance to chemosystematics, chemical ecology and biological activity **Phytochemistry,** v. 64, p. 385-393 26, 2003.

KIM, J. H.; CHOI, S. K.; LIM, W. J.; CHANG, H. I. Protective effect of astaxanthin produced by Xanthophyllomyces dendrorhous mutant on indomethacin-induced gastric mucosal injury in rats. **J Microbiol Biotechnol**, v. 14, p. 996-1003, 2004.

LEE, J. Y.; WOO, E.;KANG, K. W. Inhibition of lipopolysaccharide- inducible nitric oxide synthase expression by Verbascoside through blocking of AP-1 activation. **J Ethnopharmacol**, v. 97, p. 561-566, 2005.

LIU, M. J.; LI, J. X.; GUO, H. Z.; LEE, K. M.; QIN, L.; CHAN, K. M. The effects of verbascoside on plasma lipid peroxidation level and erythrocyte membrane fluidity during immobilization in rabbits: a time course study. **Life Sci**, v. 73, p. 883-892, 2003.

LORENZI, H.; MATOS, F. J. A. **Plantas medicinais no Brasil: nativa e exóticas.** 2 ed. Sao Paulo: Instituto Plantarumde Estudos da Flora Ltda,

2008. p. 487.

MAHLKE, J. D. *Buddleja thyrsoides* LAM.: **Morphoanatomical, phytochemical and biological study**. 118 f. Dissertation (Master's Degree in Pharmaceutical Sciences) - Health Science Center, Federal University of Santa Maria, Rio Grande do Sul, 2007.

ODONTUYA, G.; HOULT, J. R. S.; HOUGHTON, P. J. Structure-activity relation ship for anti-inflammatory effect of luteolin and its derived glycosides. **Phytother Res**, v. 19, p. 782-786, 2005.

OLIVEIRA, D. M. S. de. **Phytochemical study and biological activities of the plant species *Buddleja stachyoides* Cham. & Schltdl. (Scrophulariaceae)**.100 f. Dissertation (Master's Degree in Pharmaceutical Sciences) - Health Sciences Sector. Federal University of Paranà, Curitiba, 2012.

OLIVEIRA, D. M. S. de; MIGUEL, M. D.; KALEGARI, M.; MIGUEL, O. G.; MOREIRA, T. F. Isolation of verbacoside and validation of an analytical method for standardization of the crude extract of the aerial parts of *Buddleja stachyoides* Cham. & Schltdl. (Scrophulariaceae). **Quim Nova**, v. 37, n. 2, 344-348, 2014.

PIAO, M. S.; KIM, M.; LEE, D. G.;PARK, Y.; HAHM, K.; MOON, Y.; WOO, E. Antioxidative Constituents from *Buddleia officinalis*. **Arch Pharm Res**, v. 26, n. 6, p. 453-457, 2003.

RIBANI, M.; BOTTOLI, C. B. G.; COLLINS, C. H.; JARDIM, I. C. S. F.; MELO, L. F. C. **Quim Nova,** v. 27, p. 771, 2004.

SOUZA, V.C. 2010. Scrophulariaceae in Lista de Espécies da Flora do Brasil. Rio de Janeiro Botanical Garden. Available at: <http://floradobrasil.jbrj.gov.br/2010/FB014541>. Accessed on: May 23, 2011.

VERTUANI, S.; BEGHELLI, E.; SCALAMBRA, E.; MALISARDI, G. COPETTI, S.; DAL TOSO, R.; BALDISSEROTTO, A.; MANFREDINI, S Activity and

Stability Studies of Verbascosideo, a Novel Antioxidant, in Dermo-Cosmetic and Pharmaceutical Topical Formulations. **Molecules**, v. 16, p. 7068-7080, 2011.

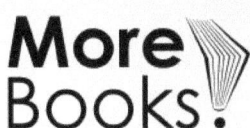
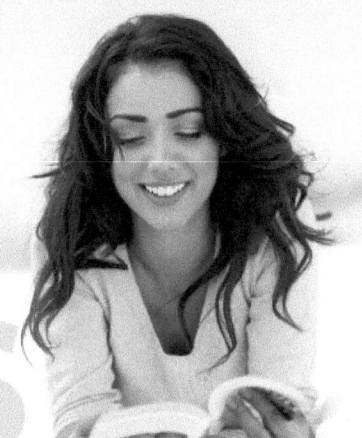

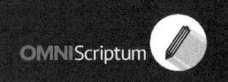

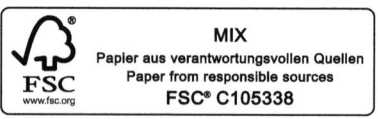
Printed by Books on Demand GmbH, Norderstedt / Germany